QUALITY ASSURANCE PRIMER
Improving Health Care Outcomes
and Productivity

by:

Patricia Curran Ostrow
John W. Williamson
Barbara E. Joe

i

Library of Congress Cataloging in Publication Data
Ostrow, Patricia Curran,
    Quality assurance primer.

    Bibliography: pp. 83-87
    Includes Index.
    1. Medical care--Quality control.   2. Medical
care--Evaluation.   3. Quality assurance.   I. Williamson, John W.,   II. Joe, Barbara E.,
III.--Title. [DNLM: 1. Quality assurance, Health
care. 2. Efficiency. W84.1 085q]
RA399.A1087   1983   362.1'028'7   83-2701
ISBN 0-910317-10-0

Cover by Corita Kent

ACKNOWLEDGMENTS

The authors wish to thank Sue Ann Ketchum for her unflagging efforts in coordinating this project and typing the manuscript.

We are especially indebted to one of our authors, John W. Williamson, not only for originating health accounting, the quality assurance approach described here, but for providing the originals which -- with his permission and minor adaptations -- have formed the basis for the illustrations, meeting agendas, tables, and forms found in this book.

TABLE OF CONTENTS

LIST OF TABLES AND FIGURES

Tables

Figures

CHAPTER I

WHY THIS BOOK?

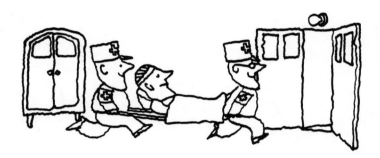

*Quality assurance should be part of health care treat-
ment from its inception. To do this, practitioners
and students need only retool their problem resolution
skills.*

I. WHY THIS BOOK?

Ninety percent of occupational therapy curriculum directors, responding to a 1981 survey, reported that quality assurance, as an element of The American Occupational Therapy Association's *Standards of Practice,* was presented in their teaching program. Many felt their students should learn even more about this important topic. The majority currently spend from 1-15 hours in class teaching quality assurance and expect their students to spend the same number of hours outside of class. All indicated they would welcome teaching aids such as study and lecture outlines, case examples, and manuals. This manual is designed to meet some of these needs, providing the essentials for teacher and student to build on. It is also intended as an introduction to quality assurance or as a refresher for the practicing health professional.

This book can be used in a variety of ways -- as a lecture guide, assigned reading, or an outline for students coming together for a quality assurance study. It is recommended that students learning about the subject engage in an actual study since the process is best learned by firsthand participation. One group of students applied the quality assurance process to their own educational program, focusing on improving personal attainment of knowledge. Their study is described in Chapter V. The goal of this book is to provide readers enough step-by-step detail to conduct an actual quality assurance study, but, for those unable to do so, it is also designed to offer a basic overview. In addition, although it is addressed mainly to occupational therapists, other health professionals should find this manual useful.

Quality assurance sharpens practitioners' problem-solving skills and stimulates creativity in patient care. The health accounting approach to quality assurance presented here focuses on improving health, economic, or societal benefits, such as enhancing patient outcomes, increasing productivity, and containing costs. Health accounting is a strategy that helps integrate many different quality assurance methods.

Health accounting has a proven record of achievement. It has highlighted situations, such as those where patients are not taking medication or using equipment as prescribed, where they do not understand the treatment plan and their role in it, or where medical records have been incomplete, resulting in missed diagnoses (see Williamson, 1982b, Chapter 10). After improvement actions to remedy these situations, patients' health and functioning has markedly improved. As added bonuses, practitioners' satisfaction often increases, while paperwork diminishes and productivity rises. Consumer input to help identify problems in patient care is a unique aspect of health accounting, which further contributes to its success. Finally, health accounting produces easily understandable documentation of the effectiveness of occupational therapy and other health care services.

This *Quality Assurance Primer* begins with a history and definitions, then goes into the stages of health accounting, including details, such as meeting agendas, for conducting a study. An example based on an actual student study is included, complete with sample forms. A final glossary, reference list, and index completes the book.

This book is intended to provide students, teachers, and professionals in a variety of health care disciplines with the basic tools for making their own contribution to the growing body of knowledge and practice in this field. This manual is a stepping stone to *Health Accounting for Quality Assurance* (Williamson, et al., 1981, copyright The American Occupational Therapy Association, Inc.), where a second type of study design opens the way to analysis of a greater range of health care problems, including poor referral patterns.

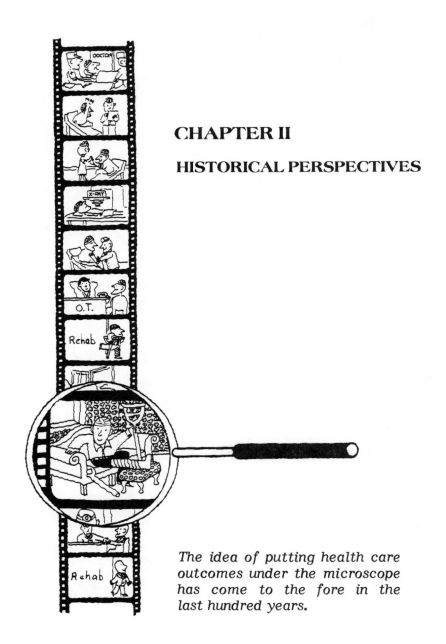

CHAPTER II

HISTORICAL PERSPECTIVES

The idea of putting health care outcomes under the microscope has come to the fore in the last hundred years.

II. HISTORICAL PERSPECTIVES

The Value of Health Care

The occupational therapy department in a rehabilitation center became concerned that patients were not motivated because they did not fully accept or understand treatment goals. The staff was able to increase the number of patients who understood short-term rehabilitation goals from 37 percent to 100 percent. It was also able to increase patient preparedness for discharge and satisfaction with health care team efforts to set mutual goals (Good, 1981).

In another facility, the occupational therapy department of a community hospital was able to increase the percentage of lumbar disc patients referred for back conservation education from 17 percent to 77 percent in a period of just two-and-a-half months (Kuntavanish, 1980).

Was some sort of magic formula dispensed or were highpowered experts brought in to achieve these results? No, for the first example it was simply a matter of applying the procedures described in this book. The second example used a study design described in *Health Accounting for Quality Assurance*. The investment of time and money was judged by all to be justified because of the improved patient care. Not only that, but the occupational therapists participating in the effort experienced an increase in work satisfaction which boosted their morale. Measuring and increasing the benefits of health care, as was done here, is the central purpose of quality assurance.

The idea of benefit is assumed in health care. Positive results and improvements beyond the ordinary course of events are implicit in health care intervention. While predictions are difficult for individual patients, there needs to be some notion of the efficacy and effectiveness of treatment for groups of patients as a whole. If the majority of patients fail to derive the expected benefits, then health care professionals need to know why. Their expectations may be unrealistic or procedures may need revision. Unless health care can stand up to this kind of self-scrutiny, the billions of dollars spent on health care, the tons of pills, bandages, splints, and equipment -- not to mention the efforts of many thousands of workers from orderlies on up -- may well be wasted.

Someone engaged in manufacturing cars or growing food produces a tangible product whose value is readily apparent to the user, who willingly parts with hard cash to purchase it. Sometimes the aggregate need is satisfied and a surplus is generated. But the basic value, which is in the product, is governed by market forces.

In health care, the product is less readily apparent and payment is largely indirect, through insurance or government reimbursement. People seeking health care presume they will benefit, though sometimes their expectations are unrealistic, "I will be cured," "I'll be able to walk again," "My pain will disappear." In fact, these results may not be achieved. Yet other benefits may accrue as products of health care activities, less concrete than a car or a bushel of corn, but no less important. Just what these benefits are, how to define, measure, and increase them, is what quality assurance is all about.

In ancient times, the value of health care, the good that flowed from the laying on of hands and the pronouncements of healers derived from the latters' exalted or magical status. If a healer told a sick man to cover himself with leeches or burn incense, it was done, no questions asked.

Some of this traditional aura still pervades health care, in the sacred doctor-patient relationship or the ready acceptance of the authority of health care practitioners. Health care is art as well as science, an expression of caring about a suffering person not amenable to exact scrutiny or measurement. Empathy, caring, and art all have their place in health care. Indeed, the patient's trust in the practitioner is an important element in the healing process.

Health Care Under Scrutiny

Nevertheless, there has been another, complementary strain running throughout health care, pragmatic, practical, and objective, rooted in the scientific revolution. Harvey, Willis, and other 16th century physicians shocked their contemporaries by dissecting the human body, learning about its components firsthand. In the 19th century, Florence Nightingale revolutionized medical thinking by looking systematically at results comparing military hospitals' rates of morbidity. Through her intervention, mortality in the Scutari military hospitals during the Crimean War dropped from 42 percent to 2.2 percent (Huxley, 1975, p. 117). And early in this century, Abraham Flexner stunned the medical community with his devastating critique of hospital conditions and methods of medical education (Flexner, 1910).

It was a logical passage from awareness of body parts and components of hospital treatment to the idea that the health care system itself could be systematically dissected. The first attempts at measuring health care quality were crude: did the patient live or die? But by 1912, E. A. Codman, a physician and surgery professor at Massachusetts General Hospital, had decided to attempt a more systematic evaluation.

Codman founded his own hospital and instituted "end-result" assessment to improve health care. He abstracted each case history, then re-evaluated every patient a year or more after hospitalization, classifying the results as satisfactory or unsatisfactory, assigning the latter to the following categories: diagnostic error, inadequate technical skills, poor surgical judgment, inadequate equipment or care, the disease process, and patient noncompliance (Codman, 1914).

Quality Assurance Comes of Age

Spurred by the Flexner Report and Codman's example, the American College of Surgeons inaugurated an accreditation effort in 1918, which has evolved into the program of The Joint Commission on Accreditation of Hospitals (JCAH) of today (Ostrow, 1983a).

With the advent of Medicare and Medicaid -- Federal programs of health care cost reimbursement for the elderly, poor, and disabled -- JCAH's accreditation process became the preferential route for hospitals to demonstrate their eligibility for government reimbursement. The Joint Commission on Accreditation of Hospitals has a detailed *Accreditation Manual for Hospitals* and a companion *QA Guide* to help hospitals meet standards of care. The *Accreditation Manual* calls for "an ongoing quality assurance program that includes effective mechanisms for reviewing and evaluating patient care, as well as an appropriate response to findings" (The Joint Commission on Accreditation of Hospitals, 1981, p. 151). The *QA Guide* outlines the steps required in quality assurance and describes various acceptable assessment methods, including the approach taken here which meets all JCAH requirements (The Joint Commission on Accreditation of Hospitals, 1980).

The Joint Commission on Accreditation of Hospitals specifically requires that rehabilitation personnel, including occupational therapists, "participate in the review and evaluation of the quality and appropriateness of care," and that each clinical discipline be "responsible for identifying and resolving problems related to patient care, administering or coordinating the overall quality assurance program." (The Joint Commission on Accreditation of Hospitals, 1981, pp. 165, 153. For a detailed discussion of the quality assurance standards of The Joint Commission on Accreditation of Hospitals and how they apply to occupational therapy, see Ostrow, 1983b.)

For the past decade, occupational therapists have supported quality assurance activities. Since 1978, The American Occupational Therapy Association's *Standards of Practice* have recognized the need for occupational therapists to "systematically review the quality, including outcomes, of their services, using predetermined criteria reflecting professional consensus and recent developments in research and theory" (The American Occupational Therapy Assocciation, Inc., 1978).

Health care accountability, whether established by JCAH standards or professional ethics, is here to stay. Rising health care specialization and sophistication, growing consumer awareness, and mushrooming costs — along with scrutiny by third party payors and criticisms of poor outcomes and unnecessary procedures — all have increased pressures to assure treatment is meeting intended objectives.

Quality assurance supplements credentialing, certification, and licensing in maintaining health care standards by translating them into action measures. For health care practitioners, quality assurance means looking at health care processes and outcomes to see if they are actually achieving intended goals. For patients and their families, quality assurance can spell the difference between a desirable and an unwanted result, bringing about enhanced well-being, and usually, savings of time, effort and money. For the public, which foots the bill for health insurance and public assistance, quality assurance can mean reduced dependency and stretching of health care dollars.

Quality assurance, as described in the health accounting approach used in this book, is antithetical to the usual stereotype of evaluation or regulation. It is not government or another outside entity breathing down the necks of practitioners, telling them how to perform in their profession. Rather, it is facilities and practitioners evaluating and motivating themselves, according to standards they set -- but with regard to the literature and generally accepted practice. Quality assurance is an ongoing process, integrated with the whole of health care practice, not evaluation imposed from outside. Its practitioners become skillful as change agents, acting as "levers" to dramatically improve care, with the documentation to show it. Quality assurance lends dynamism and a sense of movement to health care practice.

CHAPTER III

DEFINITIONS AND DISTINCTIONS

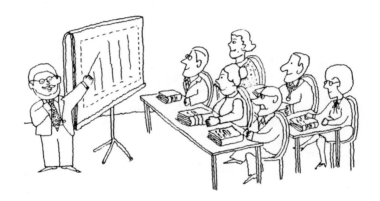

Health accounting is a quality assurance strategy.

III. DEFINITIONS AND DISTINCTIONS

Quality Assurance Defined

Quality assurance, an evaluation system that focuses on identifying and resolving important health care problems, is an obscure term to many health care professionals. Although its roots are ancient, it is a relatively new addition to the health care lexicon and not yet a household word. Just what is quality assurance? Quality assurance falls somewhere between the subjective, emotive judgment of an artist about his latest painting and the exacting, computer monitored quality control of a pharmaceutical assembly line. Both are judgments, but of a very different kind.

Health care clients are not prepackaged products, but neither are their problems totally unique. A practitioner approaches them afresh, yet drawing on experience distilled from similar situations. Every treatment program is a problem-solving exercise balancing both individual and common concerns. The practitioner identifies the individual patient's problem and does something about it.

Quality assurance goes a step further by asking and answering the question for a group of patients with a similar health problem: did our action have the expected effect and to what extent? If not, what else can we do? Is this level of care appropriate, or could it be offered at a "less intensive" level? Are the clients benefitting as much as possible and is the benefit being achieved as quickly and inexpensively as possible? Cost containment is just one type of quality assurance objective. Quality assurance (QA for short) is ongoing, objective, and improvement-oriented. (A further discussion of quality assurance in health care and quality as related to occupational therapy can be found in the 6th edition of *Willard and Spackman's Occupational Therapy*, see Chapter 43, "Quality Assurance: Improving Therapy Outcomes," Hopkins, et al., 1983.)

Quality Assurance Vis-A-Vis
Research and Program Evaluation

For health care practitioners who find the idea of "research" intimidating, it is comforting to learn that quality assurance is something different. There are basic similarities, of course. Both research and quality assurance assume laws of cause and effect, both may measure the same things in a similar way, and findings of either may complement the other. But, whereas research -- at least in the classical experimental mode -- is concerned with unearthing new knowledge, learning what is, and factual conclusions generalizable to other settings, quality assurance is a decision-making tool concerned with not only what is, but what should be, and achieving change within a particular care setting. Research is involved in corroborating theory, whereas quality assurance measures goals set against goals reached.

Politics and local contingencies, which are purged in research, play an acknowledged role in quality assurance. Quality assurance has no control groups; the standard against which activity is measured is set by the practitioners themselves. Research may be long-term, whereas a quality assurance study usually lasts from three to nine months (Holzemer, 1980).

Quality assurance, although it is not the same as research, does draw on research findings. In fact, a literature search should be part of any quality assurance study.

An example of a research study with implications for occupational therapy involved a group of 307 elderly stroke patients, half of whom received occupational therapy in a specialized stroke unit, while the other half were cared for in medical units. Almost half of the latter also received occupational therapy, but often on a delayed basis. The stroke unit patients, who all received occupational therapy promptly upon admission, were discharged an average of 20 days earlier than medical unit patients and 60 days after discharge were found to be functioning significantly better on activities of daily living (ADL) tasks (Garraway, 1980). Literature findings of this type, could appropriately inspire a health accounting study concerned with full and timely referral of stroke patients to occupational therapy.

Though research findings are important to health care progress, their significance should not be exaggerated. Treatment cannot always wait until relevant research is available. Furthermore, research findings often have a narrower range than practice, applying to a set of circumstances not always duplicated in real life. Quality assurance does not have these drawbacks, although its generalizability is less.

Quality assurance's relationship to research is one of complementarity; each has a role to play in improving health care. And, in the absence of relevant research, quality assurance draws on the group judgments of health care providers that represent a pool of knowledge and experience (see Williamson, 1975 and 1979).

Quality assurance is also closely related to program evaluation that regularly assesses how well a health care program achieves its goals. The Commission on Accreditation of Rehabilitation Facilities (CARF) requires program evaluation and amply describes the process in a set of manuals (Commission on Accreditation of Rehabilitation Facilities, May 1976, November 1976, July 1977, January 1979, December 1979, and February 1980). The scope of program evaluation is broad and encompasses both success and failure. Quality assurance differs from program evaluation by limiting its focus to specific problems in patient care, that is to particular care-giving activities practitioners feel have a large potential for improving outcomes. Quality assurance is thus in concert with the more global approach of program evaluation. But, although there is a close alliance, program evaluation and quality assurance take place independently of one another.

Health Accounting

The approach to quality assurance presented in this manual is called health accounting. It has been chosen as a comprehensive strategy for quality assurance because it has been successfully field tested in more than 80 studies. Health accounting provides self-correcting feedback mechanisms, much as a car speedometer warns us to slow down when we exceed the speed limit. It also encompasses a wide range of factors, including values and goals of both providers and consumers. Many quality assurance mechanisms focus on the structure and process of care, thus relying on "inductive" reasoning, which infers acceptable outcomes when appropriate management processes and structures are present. Health accounting emphasizes "deductive" reasoning, trying to identify correctable structures and procedures when unacceptable outcomes are found, as shown in Figure A.

Figure A
Quality Assurance Cycle

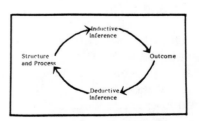

Health care outcomes refer to any characteristic of patient, health problem, or provider that results from health care received (or withheld) at any given point in time. Note that an outcome can be measured at any time in the treatment program or even after discharge.

While admittedly, the dividing line between ends and means is not always clearcut, looking at results generally has several advantages. Ends, by definition, are the final products of actions evaluated as either desirable or undesirable. If ends are desired, the treatment actions related to them are substantiated. If the ends are not desired, those processes can be revised until appropriate achievable outcomes are attained.

Looking at outcomes is more direct than looking at health care processes, since approved methods may not actually produce desired results. Treatment processes can be most economically evaluated according to their outcomes. Evaluation which short-cuts directly to outcomes avoids excessive speculation and debate over whether or not to employ particular treatment modalities. Outcomes measurement tends to be quicker and more cost effective than monitoring the myriad of health care treatment processes.

A discussion of means and ends is not a mere philosophical exercise. It lies at the heart of health accounting, which basically asks: are we achieving our desired health, economic, or societal goals? If not, why not? If the reasons are correctable, let's change the care. If the reasons are not correctable, let's change the goals.

For the theoretical underpinnings of quality assessment and improvement, we are indebted to Avedis Donabedian, MD, MPH, Professor of Medical Care Organization at the University of Michigan School of Public Health (Donabedian, 1969, 1980, 1982). Donabedian defines quality health care as "that kind of care which is expected to maximize..... patient welfare after one has taken account of the balance of gains and losses (health benefits and risks) that attend the process of care in all its parts" (Donabedian, 1980, pp. 5-6). Among the losses or risks, Donabedian includes cost.

While Donabedian has set the stage, the practical, operational method of quality assurance designated as health accounting was originated by John W. Williamson, MD, Professor of Health Services Administration and International Health at Johns Hopkins School of Hygiene and Public Health. This approach was developed, tested, and taught over the past 15 years in a variety of settings, some as far away as the Netherlands. The American Occupational Therapy Association has also field-tested this approach (The American Occupational Therapy Association, Inc., 1980).

In a 1978 assessment of health accounting studies, four out of five projects achieved statistically significant improvements. Studies also generated financial savings that more than offset their initial cost (Williamson, 1978c). But, despite this proven record, outcomes review is regarded apprehensively by some professionals who prefer the security of process review, such as documentation, and fear what outcomes measures might reveal. There may also be pessimism about improving outcomes. Participation in a health accounting study usually erases these concerns, as soon as worthwhile improvements become apparent.

Health accounting is a way first of identifying and measuring a problem, next taking action to solve this problem, then measuring to see if the improvement action actually produced the desired solution. If not, a new remedy is tried.

There are three considerations in health accounting -- efficacy, effectiveness, and efficiency. Efficacy is the result of a particular health intervention under ideal, controlled circumstances. Thus, a given medication, properly administered, might show almost 100 percent efficacy in controlling a given condition in laboratory trials. But the effectiveness of the medication in a particular treatment program might be drastically lower. Effectiveness refers to the results of care in a specific department or facility. Finally, there is the efficiency of a given technique in terms of both time and cost.

The reader needs to become comfortable with the concepts of efficacy, effectiveness, and efficiency, and with the rest of the specialized health accounting vocabulary that provides useful short-cuts in talking and thinking about this subject. Most of the terms used in health accounting will be discussed in subsequent sections. A total compilation can be found in the Glossary.

Productivity and Cost Containment

With spiraling health costs and disturbing reports of waste -- or even damage -- resulting from health care intervention, efforts are being made to improve health care quality without increasing costs. Efficiency, as used in health accounting, embodies the notion of cost containment or reduction, and better utilization of scarce medical resources. Health care practitioners can, through quality assurance, improve health care outcomes, and learn to do so in the shortest time with the least possible expenditure of staff effort and equipment.

It is difficult for a beginner in health accounting to study effectiveness and cost simultaneously. It is therefore advisable in beginning studies to hold one or the other constant. The first study objective is to improve care outcomes; a subsequent study could tackle the problem of maintaining the improved level of care, while at the same time reducing costs and/or increasing productivity. Methods of increasing productivity without decreasing quality, such as use of group techniques, and family or volunteer helpers, and appropriate delegation to certified occupational therapy assistants, might be tested in an occupational therapy department. Always there is the question: Is this the least expensive way to provide what these patients need?

Services given or devices provided where they are not used or needed are obviously unproductive. For example, a rehabilitation facility learned that most patients were not using their adaptive devices after going home. Here, patient education about use of adaptive devices needs to be revised or better post-discharge follow-up designed.

The value of lives saved and disabilities prevented cannot easily be expressed in dollars. However, measurable cost savings can be derived from shortening hospital stays, reducing absences from work, and decreasing need for future hospitalization. "The best care at the least cost" needs to be the axiom of health care professionals and health accounting is one avenue for achieving this. (See Williamson, 1982a for more on this topic.)

The Paperwork Bugaboo

One of the biggest apprehensions about health accounting is that it will not increase efficiency, but will actually add to the paperwork and reporting burden, stealing precious time from patient care. Health accounting, especially a first study, does take extra time and planning, but subsequent studies can be readily blended into regular program operations. Skills are learned that enhance total care and staff morale and often generate new efficiencies, thus more than compensating for the time and effort expended. Indeed, one of the central objectives of health accounting is to reduce costs and make operations more efficient. This includes keeping health accounting studies themselves "lean" in terms of paperwork.

A health accounting study in a psychiatric facility tackled the paperwork monster head-on and found it to be a paper tiger. The study applied health accounting directly to the problem of excess staff time spent in documenting health care services. The study proved to be successful in consolidating and simplifying reporting methods, decreasing documentation time by four hours per week per therapist, thus freeing this time for patient care (Ostrow and Kaufman, 1981). The most important aspect of this study was the fact that health outcomes were not impaired by the increase in efficiency; in fact, they were enhanced, according to a parallel study. The effects of such an increase in productivity can be profound, especially when multiplied by the several therapists usually found in an occupational therapy department.

Achievable Benefits Not Achieved (ABNA)

A key concept in health accounting is ABNA, achievable benefits not achieved. ABNA represents lost opportunity, potential not realized. In health care, ABNA can spell the difference between life and death, or between optimal vs. marginal functioning. We are not concerned here with new treatments, but with full application of already-proven modalities. ABNA is a shorthand way of referring simultaneously to the efficacy (achievable benefits) and effectiveness (actually achieved benefits) of treatment.

In a health accounting study of patients with hypertension, 36 percent were out-of-control (blood pressure abnormal) compared with a pre-set standard of 5 percent. Since hypertension is readily controllable by medication, this indicated an area for improvement action. After a patient education program, the percentage of patients whose blood pressure was out-of-control dropped to 19 percent; an improvement, but still considered too high, given the life-threatening course of the uncontrolled disease. Further action brought the uncontrolled level to 13 percent (Williamson, 1975).

25

Action was still called for. But the main lessons of the study were clear. First, just because a treatment with proven efficacy is prescribed does not mean success will be automatic. Second, systematic action can improve outcomes. Finally, in this situation, the well-known benefits of hypertension medication were not being achieved, but were achievable, resulting in high ABNA.

Maximum Acceptable Standards (MAS)

This brings us to the related concept of maximum acceptable standards (MAS). MAS refers to the highest percentage of patients whose health problem can be expected (or tolerated) to be out-of-control, given optimal treatment. Most standards have a positive valence. But in health accounting, where the focus is on improvement potential, the standard refers to a negative. The MAS is a maximum level of acceptable deficiency. With MAS, the goal is to reach near to or below the maximum acceptable standard for noncontrol. This "out-of-control" maximum is the counterpart to an "in-control" percentage. Thus, an MAS of 15 percent would mean 85 percent in control. Because quality assurance focuses on improving problem areas, a maximum level of acceptable problem noncontrol is needed. This is what the MAS provides.

The MAS is set in advance by the team studying a particular health care problem. If preliminary data show that, under existing treatment conditions, the number of patients with a health problem out-of-control meets the MAS or is even lower, then no improvement action is called for because the standard is being achieved. If, on the other hand, there is a big gap between the actual number out-of-control and the MAS, this would indicate an area for consideration of improvement action. Health accounting deals with reducing problems, hence the importance of measuring noncontrol.

Both to illustrate MAS and to provide some insight into real-life: in one study of stroke patients in a rehabilitation program, staff established 5 percent as the upper level of patient failure to know the objectives of treatment. This meant, conversely, that 95 percent of patients could be expected to be able to communicate their treatment goals, leaving an MAS of 5 percent. However, preliminary investigation, based on 15 patient questionnaires, showed 63 percent unable to state their treatment goals, falling far short of the MAS and indicating a need for improvement action. Staff felt the patients would not be fully involved with treatment efforts if they did not know the goals. Improvement action included writing down the goals for patients in layman's language and displaying them clearly in the patient's room, on a blackboard, then repeating the goals using the same language during patient treatments. All staff were to refer to each goal as it related to any treatment given and in patient/family conferences. All families received written copies of the goals.

The results during the first reanalysis of the problem seemed beneficial. The noncontrol rate, based on patients' inability to state their treatment goals, was reduced from 63 percent to 0, well below the MAS of 5 percent (Good, 1981).

Although this seems to be a very striking improvement, and well may indicate a real trend, the sample for the post-improvement analysis was small.

The post-improvement questionnaire was administered by a student to only five patients due to a low patient census during the student's three-month affiliation. A larger sample would have been needed to place confidence in the improvement. Further case analysis is necessary in this example, but the student's study provided valuable training for her and assisted the center in their quality assurance activities.

Skills Development Exercise I -- Definitions

As a hypothetical case, a new hand splint has been found that, in controlled trials, prevents wrist drop in 98 percent of stroke patients if worn daily. In clinic A, prevention is being achieved in only 50 percent of cases. Staff feel a 90 percent prevention rate is possible in their clinic and that 10 percent is the upper limit of noncontrol. There are two variants of the splint, with equal results in clinical trials, one of which costs 25 percent less than the other.

1. Describe this situation in terms of efficacy, effectiveness, and efficiency.

2. What is the MAS?

(Answers in Appendix A)

The terms discussed and defined in this chapter will prove useful in the health accounting process, described in the next chapter.

CHAPTER IV

STAGES OF HEALTH ACCOUNTING

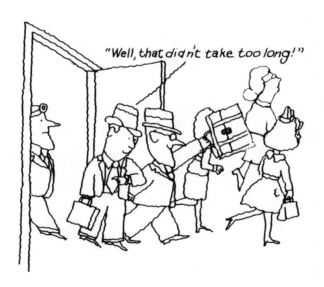

Health accounting can be easily mastered by health professionals.

IV. STAGES OF HEALTH ACCOUNTING

There are five stages in health accounting, though content will vary according to the particular study and facility. These stages are: (1) priority setting, concerned with selecting a topic or problem for study; (2) initial outcome assessment, which designs the study and confirms (or negates) the existence of the problem; (3) definitive assessment and improvement planning, which refines the problem and maps out the improvement action; (4) improvement action, that is, actually implementing the improvement(s) planned in Stage 3; and (5) outcome reassessment, testing the results of the improvement action. Figure B shows the stages of health accounting.

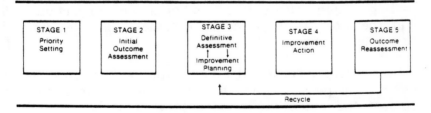

Figure B
Stages of Health Accounting

This chapter will first generally describe, then specifically outline each of the five stages of health accounting, providing enough detail to conduct a health accounting study. After the general description, a specific outline of steps to follow will be shown in italics. Chapter V will then give an example, based on an actual student study, illustrating these stages.

Stage 1 -- Priority Setting

The first stage of health accounting is to identify important, solvable problems in patient care whose resolutions will be worth the effort/money required to study and remedy them. Judgments about importance, solvability, and cost effectiveness are based on structured group decision making. This is done in a multidisciplinary meeting, called the priority setting meeting, that includes a patient representative.

All parties may not initially agree on what constitutes an important problem. The meeting allows a systematic discussion of individual perceptions so that problems whose solution could significantly improve patient outcomes will be identified for study.

The problem chosen for study and remedy via health accounting must not only be important, but also solvable within current parameters of knowledge, feasibility, and practicality. Solvability is usually translated into the shorthand ABNA (achievable benefits not achieved). That is, the solution is known and tested (or, in the absence of hard data, experienced professionals agree on its efficacy), but successful outcomes are not being fully realized in the given setting. High ABNA is an indication of importance and therefore is a factor to consider when deciding to pursue a study.

Cost effectiveness falls under the rubric of efficiency. Expensive remedies need to be measured against the objective to be achieved. It might well be that the same effort expended in another area would have a greater return. In sum, which achievable benefits (efficacy) are being achieved (effectiveness) at what cost (efficiency)?

Finally, the problem selected for a quality assurance study must occur with sufficient frequency to permit the study to take place and make improvement worthwhile. All these conditions must be met to identify good health accounting study topics.

For instance, in Stage 1, a health accounting study might be initiated in the occupational therapy department of a hospital by the quality assurance coordinator of that department, a role that could be rotated among the senior staff. The coordinator issues a memo to a preselected, multidisciplinary team of five to thirteen members, at least half of whom are occupational therapists since it is their department that is being studied. This team, called priority team, usually includes at least one person representing each of the following: administration, physicians, and consumers. Other relevant health care practitioners (nurse, physical therapist) should also be included. This multidisciplinary approach is in keeping with JCAH standards, which call for "the participation of both physicians and other health professionals in the same quality assessment activities." (Joint Commission on Accreditation of Hospitals, 1981, p. 152.)

The priority setting meeting takes place using a modified nominal group process. It has been found that such a structured group technique generates more and better ideas and solutions in a shorter time than simple open dialogue (Van de Ven, et al., 1971). The nominal technique is described more fully by Delbecq (Delbecq, et al., 1975).

This process should generate enough topics for six to twelve months of quality assurance activity, with any one study scheduled to last not more than nine months. Not all topics require a full study to resolve them; some respond well to individual action, once identified. Final study topic selection may require a stamp of approval at medical and administrative levels. Involvement of these levels early in the planning of the study is recommended to ensure support for later improvement actions.

This has been an overview of Stage 1. The following is a step-by-step guide for actually conducting Stage 1.

Outline for Stage 1 -- Priority Setting

(Note: blank forms and additional elaboration are available in Williamson, et al., 1981, from which this guide is adapted. Experienced practitioners can modify the format, but, for first timers, it is recommended that this guide, including time limits, be closely observed.)

Preparation

A few weeks before the scheduled priority setting meeting, it is helpful if the quality assurance coordinator sends a memo to priority team participants, telling them the time and place of the meeting and its purpose: namely to identify high-priority problems in health care. The team should be multidisciplinary and contain from five to thirteen members; larger groups are strongly discouraged because they are too unwieldy for this process. Beginners usually do better with small groups.

The quality assurance coordinator normally serves as Stage 1 facilitator. He or she may be a full-time person appointed for an entire institution or may be assigned from a department to conduct a department-wide study. The first-time coordinator/facilitator should select a group size and composition that seems comfortable. When planning the team composition, try to choose people who can work well together in a group.

Priority Setting Meeting

In health accounting, the discussion leader is called a facilitator because he/she is not a leader in the usual sense of guiding a meeting in a predetermined direction. Usually the health accounting facilitator is not a participant at all, but someone to keep the discussion moving through the agenda in an orderly and timely manner. The content of the meeting is fashioned by the group members, who should all have an equal opportunity to participate.

Before the meeting, it is recommended that the facilitator review the nominal group process. It is quite different from a spontaneous or social group. Verbal interaction is limited to specified times within specified time limits.

Briefly, here are the major steps in the nominal group process: after a brief introduction, the facilitator asks each member, working alone, to write down ideas for study. A question to guide their thinking is written on the flipchart. Next, going around the room, the facilitator writes down each idea, about 25 (see Table 1 for sample ideas). The ideas are clarified in brief discussion, then weighted for a combination of importance, solvability, and cost effectiveness by individual ballot, on a scale from one to five (five representing high priority). The group then analyzes and discusses some of the topics based on ballot results and finally re-weights the topics.

Table 1

Illustrative Quality Assurance Topics
Developed by Structured Group Process

A. Follow-up evaluation by occupational therapists of return to major life activity of male post-myocardial infarction patients 40 to 50 years of age.

B. Group counseling by occupational therapists for better self-care and use of activity by adults with chronic heart disease.

C. Appropriate referral to occupational therapy of the patient with lumbar disc derangement and displacement.

D. Better follow-up by occupational therapy of premature babies to screen for developmental lag and treat appropriately.

Facilitator's Agenda

For Priority Setting Meeting

(2 hours and 20 minutes)

Supplies needed: flipchart, masking tape, wide felt-tipped pens, forms or blank paper.

1. Introduction *(10 minutes)*

    Clarify the purpose of the meeting, go over the time-table, and make introductions on a first-name-only basis (this establishes equality within the group).

    Review ABNA; nominal group technique.

    Display and explain the three essential criteria for establishing priority problems.

    a. *Importance -- involves serious loss if not solved.*

    b. *Solvability -- care efficacy, improvement considered feasible.*

    c. *Cost effectiveness -- probable impact worth total effort.*

    Write the nominal question so all can see it: What problems in your facility, related to occupational therapy services, meet the three criteria?

2. Individual Topic Formulation *(10 minutes)*

    Pass around blank paper. Ask each team member to silently and privately list topic ideas that come to mind without prejudging or ana-

lyzing them. Each topic should encompass only one problem. Do not discuss the topics at this time.

Ask each person privately to select two topics from their list that meet the three criteria.

3. <u>Group Collation</u> *(25 minutes)*
   <u>and Discussion</u> *(10 minutes)*

   Going around the room in sequence twice (or three times if it is a small group), ask each person for an idea, then write each one on the flipchart without comment. If a topic obviously has been covered, ask for a show of hands to see if the group agrees without getting involved in discussion. Eliminate nearly identical topics, but not those with some overlap. Letter, do not number, the topics on the flipchart to avoid confusion with weighting numbers used later. Do not discuss topics during this process.

   Display all 15 to 25 topics simultaneously (usually attached to a wall with masking tape). Ask the group whether they understand each topic well enough to make an initial weighting of its importance, solvability, and cost effectiveness. Discuss topics for clarification only, no analysis or judgments at this time. Be sure everyone has the general idea, without getting involved with specifics, about what needs to be changed to improve the problem.

4. <u>Individual Topic Priority Weighting</u> *(5 minutes)*

   Provide blank paper. Each person identifies their paper by noting the last three digits of their home telephone number in the upper right hand corner. Ask each individual to weight the topics, identifying them from A to Z in the left margin of the paper. On a scale of 5 (high) to 1 (low), give an overall rating to each topic according to the three criteria above.

5. **Collation of Priority Weights** *(15 minutes)*

Facilitator collects all weighting sheets, mixes the order, and passes them around again. This allows speedy tabulation and still ensures a "blind vote." Then the leader marks the number of "votes" for each weight directly on the flipchart next to each topic. The following box is useful to record the scores:

5	4	3	2	1

Tally them as each topic is weighted

5	4	3	2	1
2	3	1	6	0

$$= (5 \times 2) + (4 \times 3)$$
$$+ (3 \times 1) + (2 \times 6)$$
$$+ (1 \times 0) = 37$$

Return rating sheets to their owners.

6. **Group Discussion and Reweighting of Topics** *(60 minutes)*

Using the three priority criteria, analyze topics with high votes, divergent votes, (a split in high and low weightings), and others if time permits). Ask: what are the strong points of each topic?

a. High votes mean high consensus and may require little discussion.

b. Divergent votes indicate controversial or unclear topics.

c. There may be combining of topics, but beware of handling more than one problem per topic.

Be sure the topic is stated so that the group's intention is clear. All topics discussed should be pinpointed, if time permits, by specifying the following:

a. *Subject/setting (identify subjects/patients involved in the problem -- age, location, sex).*

b. *Health problem characteristics. (Note what diagnoses or health deficiencies are considered in this topic -- stroke, ADL deficiency.)*

c. *Provider/facility characteristics. (list who is providing care for the problem, who needs to change -- occupational therapists, physicians, nurses).*

d. *Possible care change to improve outcomes (indicate what change is necessary to improve outcomes -- group self-care counseling by an occupational therapist, improved referrals).*

After the discussion, individually reweight topics analyzed.

7. <u>Conclusion</u> *(5 minutes)*

Collect all final weightings. Adjourn, thank participants, telling them they will be informed of final weighting and topic selection.

<u>Collation of Final Topic Weights</u>

After the priority team has adjourned, the facilitator collates the final topic weights and makes a permanent record of the results of the meeting. However, before final topic selection, the facilitator reviews each topic:

- *Is the topic understandable as stated? (If not, add a clarifying sentence.)*

- *Is it a quality assurance topic or really research? (If research, omit from the list or refer to the facility research committee, if there is one.)*

- *Can the problem be handled by individual action without a full study to bring about change? (If yes, plan appropriate individual action and follow-up to check for problem resolution. This is also an element of a quality assurance program even though improvement action is simple to achieve.)*

The results of the meeting can be circulated to participants. Resolution of problems (study topics) revealed in this meeting should be tracked and documented as part of quality assurance records useful for accreditation surveys.

Topic Selection

Though topics with the highest weight are normally selected, high priority topics are frequently forwarded to top administrators on the Quality Assurance Committee in a health care facility for their final review and concurrence before being announced. Early involvement of significant others in a facility is often essential to implementation of improvement actions necessary to improve the problem. Beginners should be careful to choose only one discrete topic and not try to assess multiple outcomes in the same study.

Notifying team members of the final topic chosen marks the end of Stage 1.

Stage 2 -- Initial Outcome Assessment

The overall purpose of Stage 2 is to clarify the nature and dimensions of the problem. It is the longest stage in terms of steps and preparation time. As with Stage 1, there will be an overview here of Stage 2, followed by a specific guide (in italics) to conducting this stage of a health accounting study.

Some preliminary activities must be concluded before the actual study can get underway in Stage 2. The study coordinator, or an assistant, searches the literature for material bearing on the chosen topic. A realistic time-frame for the search should be established. There may also be relevant data, such as the number of patients admitted annually and average length of stay, already available from the facility.

Study Team Selection and Study Design Meeting

The next step is for the quality assurance study coordinator to select the study team, usually four to five members, all having experience in the topic area. (This is not the same group as the priority selection team of Stage 1, which was larger.)

At the study design meeting, the literature findings are presented. Using a structured group process, the group will refine the problem, decide how to locate the population that will serve as the sampling pool, select a sampling technique, set the MAS, and decide whether the expected improvement justifies the money and effort to be expended.

The study design meeting will offer a chance to decide "go/no go" on the study plan. If "no go," another topic may be selected. A "go" decision indicates commitment to solving the specific problem and confidence the problem is important, solvable, and practical to solve within the constraints of time, money, and other resources.

Decision Versus Action Outcomes

During the study design meeting, a determination must be made about whether the topic is a decision or an action outcome study.

There are two types of health care outcomes and it is important to understand the difference. There are outcomes of decisions, which relate to judgments about referral, evaluation and choice of treatment procedures. Then there are outcomes of actions taken, referring to the way a decision is carried out.

Whether to refer a patient to occupational therapy, use neurodevelopmental treatment (NDT) techniques with a patient, or select independent self-care as a treatment goal are all examples of health care decisions. The decision to act or not to act results in a decision outcome, such as that patients who need occupational therapy may not be referred (or that patients who do not need occupational therapy are inappropriately referred).

Action outcomes, in turn, are the results of actually carrying out a decision, such as the process of referring to occupational therapy (Does it take three days? Are referrals lost?), the manner of providing NDT, or method of training in activities of daily living. Some health care outcomes may fall into either an action or a decision outcome, depending on where the team feels the major process problem lies. Be sure not to have a first study tackle both types of outcomes at once. (See Skills Development Exercise 2.)

Beginners in health accounting are advised to choose a clearcut action outcome study because that study design is easier to perform. It will be the only study design presented here. Those wishing to do a decision outcome study should refer to Williamson, et al., *Health Accounting for Quality Assurance,* Stage 2.

Skills Development Exercise 2
Decision Outcomes and Action Outcomes

The following exercise has been designed to help the reader learn to distinguish decision outcome from action outcome topics.

Instructions

Based on the information given below, decide whether the following problems primarily involve decision (D) or action (A) outcomes, or possibly both. For each item, circle the correct letter(s).

Problems

D   A   1.   The multidisciplinary priority team at an acute-care facility feels that certain geriatric patients could be discharged sooner if referred earlier in their hospitalization to occupational therapy for independent living skills assessment and training.

D   A   2.   Hospital staff is concerned that too many of their depression patients are not showing adequate improvement.

D   A   3.   An attending physician noticed that some patients who had hip fracture received referral to occupational therapy and physical therapy and others did not. Concern was expressed at a staff meeting that physicians appeared to have a problem in deciding whether to utilize these therapies.

D   A   4.   There is consumer concern that the education of certain cardiac patients and their families is inadequate, preventing full return to the medically feasible level of activity.

D A   5.   Rehabilitation staff is concerned that com-
            munication between disciplines is ineffec-
            tive and treatment may therefore be poorly
            coordinated.

D A   6.   Occupational therapy staff in a psychiatric
            setting felt that use of sensory integrative
            therapy was widely divergent. They felt
            that it was not clear to staff which type
            of patient should receive this therapy.

(Answers in Appendix B.)

Sample Size and Selection

   Another function of the study design meeting is
to decide on the sample size. The study sample is
intended to represent the population from which it
is drawn. For purposes of a beginning study, a final
sample of 20 to 30 subjects is sufficient. Start out
with at least 25 subjects, since a few will probably
not be available or not qualify. Be careful that you
do not lose more than 20 percent of your initial sample
or it will cease to "represent" the base population
from which it was drawn. For those with quality assurance experience, further information about the
rules governing sample size and selection techniques
is discussed elsewhere (Williamson, et al., 1981, pp. 15-29).

Sampling Method

   In addition to staying with a sample of between
20 and 30, the beginner is advised, as a matter of sim-
plicity, to use consecutive sampling, rather than random or stratified random methods. Consecutive
sampling may involve taking the first 25 or more clients
admitted, or every second or third one, until the
requisite number is obtained. If every person in the
entire population you wish to study is to be included,
then it is a universe sample. Clients may be sampled
retrospectively (in the past, after treatment has been

given, i.e., through records), concurrently (as patients presently in the hospital), or prospectively (upon admission, beginning with a specified future date).

Not only do the subjects have to be selected, but the aspects of care or functioning to be studied need to be chosen. What is it we want to measure to show that problem control has been achieved and what method will be used? For example, we might decide to ask how many patients in the sample return to work within a given time-table? How many are able to feed themselves at discharge? How many continue to use adaptive devices at home? Data can be collected directly from medical records, by observation, or through client interview, phone call, or letter (Skills Development Exercise 3 provides practice in designing an action outcome study).

Skills Development Exercise 3
Selecting Study Sample and Measuring Action Outcomes

Instructions

To measure the dimensions of each problem, (a) define the population base from which the sample would be drawn, (b) describe the sample method that would be used, (c) indicate what would be measured and when.

Topics

1. Increase early referrals to occupational therapy of stroke patients.

2. Improve the transportation of hospitalized non-ambulatory patients to occupational therapy treatments.

3. Augment the ADL program with effective stress management education for all rehabilitation patients and families.

(Answers in Appendix C.)

Study Implementation

Now the initial assessment of the problem begins. Medical records are checked, questionnaires formulated, and data collection begun. After the data is collected, it must be tabulated, reported to the study team, and fed into the existing administrative and evaluation systems of the facility. After the data display (in a graph) is prepared, Stage 2 is finished. The outline of specific steps to guide Stage 2 follows.

Outline for Stage 2 -- Initial Outcome Assessment

This stage includes selecting the study team and conducting the study design meeting. The team has four or five members, experienced in the area being studied and able to work in a group. The study design meeting has five parts, represented by the initials "IDSAW" for Introduction, Design, Simulation, Analysis, and Wrap-up. For beginners, the meeting can be split into two parts, the first consisting of "ID" and lasting about an hour, the second of "SAW," about two hours long.

The facilitator for the study design meeting may be, at times, different than the one for the priority setting meeting. For instance, the quality assurance coordinator for the whole facility may serve as the facilitator for the priority setting meeting, whereas, the Director of Occupational Therapy may be the study design meeting facilitator for an occupational therapy study. There is an advantage of continuity if they are the same person, but this is not always possible.

Facilitator's Agenda

For Study Design Meeting

(2 hours and 40 minutes)

Supplies needed: flipchart, masking tape, wide felt-tipped pens, forms or blank paper. A pocket calculator is useful.

Introduction (10 minutes)

1. *Clarify the purpose of the meeting, make introductions on a first-name basis.*

2. *Show chart (Figure C), explain Stage 2, the team role, and place of Stage 2 in the five-stage system. Overall task for Stage 2 meeting is to measure the extent of the problem identified in Stage 1.*

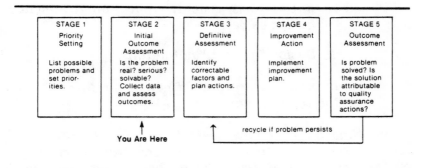

STAGE 1	STAGE 2	STAGE 3	STAGE 4	STAGE 5
Priority Setting	Initial Outcome Assessment	Definitive Assessment	Improvement Action	Outcome Assessment
List possible problems and set priorities.	Is the problem real? serious? solvable? Collect data and assess outcomes.	Identify correctable factors and plan actions.	Implement improvement plan.	Is problem solved? Is the solution attributable to quality assurance actions?

You Are Here

recycle if problem persists

Figure C
Stages in Problem Solving

3. *Review why this topic was selected; it was judged to have high ABNA (to be important, solvable, cost effective by the priority team). Review literature findings relevant to the topic.*

4. *Discuss <u>Why This Meeting</u>*

   a. *To decide the study design for Stage 2 (who, what, where, and when).*

   b. *To establish outcome standards.*

   c. *To determine feasibility of study design.*

5. *Highlight team agenda emphasizing time constraints.*

6. *Remind team that study is concerned with:*

   a. *Evaluation, not research.*

   b. *Outcomes, not processes.*

   c. *Initial assessment, not improvement action as yet.*

   d. *Design "gestalt," not details.*

7. *Review literature findings relevant to the topic, if any.*

The time allotted may seem brief, but it is important to recognize time and cost constraints on busy professionals. Field trials have shown that the suggested time limits, with occasional modifications, are reasonable. The facilitator should record decisions of the team as they are made. The Study Design Summary Form (Appendix D) was designed to serve this purpose. Such a record will assist review of the study during final wrap-up of the meeting.

Design *(50 minutes)*

1. State that the aim of this phase is to complete an initial overall outline of the study design, establishing a base for setting standards and making a first judgment on feasibility. This design skeleton will be fleshed out during simulation, the next part of the meeting.

2. _Who_ and _what_ to study

   a. Review the four factors of the study topic -- the subjects, health problem, providers, and care change to improve outcomes (see p. 39) so that the study design team understands these elements and agrees with the descriptions given by the priority team.

3. _Which_ outcome to improve; be sure this is an action outcome study.

4. _Where_ to locate subjects:

   a. Decide sampling source, will it be charts, appointment lists, other records? Consider if there are enough patients to make the Stage 2 study feasible to complete in three months.

   b. Choose sample method, either simple consecutive, systematic consecutive (every second or third), or universe sample (all patients involved).

   c. Consider if there are enough patients in three months to complete the Stage 2 data collection. (Recommended sample size, 20 to 30 subjects.)

5. *How* to measure outcomes:

    a. Define noncontrol of the problem. Sometimes it is easier to describe problem control first. To begin this task ask: How will you know when the problem is solved? What will you see when the problem is resolved? i.e., patients' ADL function compatible with ability. If you are not seeing these things, the problem is out of control, i.e., patients' ADL skills are not being used.

    b. Select objective method of assessing noncontrol.

6. *When* to conduct the study (initial estimate).

    a. Decide when to sample subjects: retrospectively, concurrently, or prospectively. Set dates.

    b. Decide when to gather data: retrospectively, concurrently, or prospectively. Set dates.

    c. Set beginning and end of study. Decide dates.

7. Decide whether this initial study seems feasible after reviewing it.

Simulation (60-90 minutes)

1. **Explain the purpose of simulation,** which is to test out the study design by mentally walking through it from start to finish.

2. **Estimate base population.** This is the population from which the sample will be drawn. It may be the total study population or only a segment that is very much "at risk"

for the problem. Estimate how many per year are in the facility population and divide by 12 for monthly average. Any data the facilitator has collected prior to the meeting is useful here.

3. *Set MAS. Review problem noncontrol and ask each participant to set the MAS initially, then again after discussion. Remember, the MAS is the maximum tolerable rate of noncontrol of the problem.*

4. *Estimate expected findings. After discussion about what the group expects to find before and after improvement action, group members note the percent of problem noncontrol they expect to find if the study were done today, as well as the expected level after improvement action.*

Analysis *(10 minutes)*

1. *State the aim of this section, which is to review the study design for continuity and feasibility, to examine the difference between the expected findings and the MAS, and to make a "go/no go" decision.*

2. *Review study design; compare MAS and expected findings.*

A small difference between the expected findings before improvement action and the MAS indicates the study may not be worth the effort. Or a small difference between the expected findings before and after improvement action means the group doesn't feel much can be achieved. Either way, it is best not to go ahead with a study topic where these differences are small.

3. *Make final "go/no go" decision.*

Wrap-up *(10 minutes)*

1. *Clarify plan for study implementation, next steps, assignment of responsibilities.*

2. *Assign responsibilities for sampling, creation of measurement instruments, if needed, data collection, and reporting.*

3. *Set date for completion of above tasks and for completion of remaining stages.*

Study Implementation

After the study design meeting, it is time to implement the study. This requires designing a questionnaire, if that is necessary, selecting the sample, and otherwise gathering the data as appropriate. Usually these tasks have already been delegated to study design team members who proceed to carry them out.

Here are some methods of data-gathering:

- *Chart review*

- *Patient interview*

- *Questionnaire*

- *Observation*

Principles of questionnaire design are as follows:

1. Know your objectives.

2. Be precise.

3. Be brief.

4. Ask one question at a time.

5. Pre-select response choices, avoiding simple "yes" and "no" or "open-ended" questions.

6. Be objective and nonjudgmental.

7. Make questions applicable to all respondents.

8. Consider question order.

9. Be thorough.

10. Be sensitive to feelings, values, and social norms of individuals being surveyed.

11. Consider tone of questions, avoid sounding patronizing or grilling. (Adapted from Williamson, 1981, pp. 50-54.)

After the data is gathered, it must be summarized and tabulated in written form. It is most easily understood if displayed in a graph (See Figure D).

Stage 3 -- Definitive Assessment and Improvement Planning

Another meeting of the study is called after the results of the Stage 2 study are in, to review the data and start planning for improvement. Of course, if the results fall within the MAS, the study stops since no improvement action is therefore indicated. For example, a study of stroke rehabilitation inpatients found them actually doing better than expected under current treatment, justifying no change in methods (Anderson, 1978). Consequently, the subsequent stages of health accounting become unnecessary. Ideally speaking, a no-problem topic should not have been studied to begin with and should have been eliminated in Stage 1.

When the data is collected, organized and displayed in a graph, Stage 2 is complete.

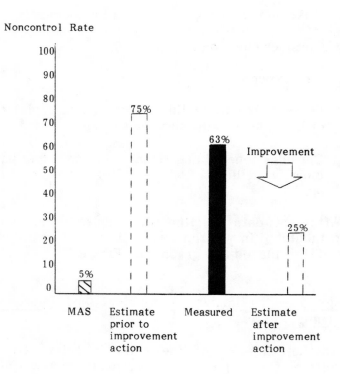

Figure D

Health Problem Noncontrol
Results of Initial Assessment

Definition of health problem noncontrol: patient (or family member) lacks knowledge of short-term rehabilitation goals.

The beauty of health accounting is that it is not a closed, rigid system. It is a problem-solving system in which a study can be stopped or revised at any stage along the way. However, in general, careful topic review means that a problem with high ABNA has been initially selected. The data will then confirm the existence of the problem, providing a base-line to assess improved status, and the study will continue on to Stage 3.

Next, the quality assurance coordinator elicits from the study team their ideas on possible correctable causes, asking the team to work individually and then share their best ideas with the group, as was done in the Priority Setting Meeting. After all the ideas are displayed, one can analyze them and do just one weighting, without striving for a "secret ballot," to save time. Causes can be categorized as patient factors (lack of understanding or cooperation), provider factors (lack of knowledge or skill), organizational factors (facility organization and procedures), and health care environment factors (legal or economic conditions, scarcity). A mini-study may be authorized to elucidate or corroborate the causes identified.

As for remedies, the question is: What needs to be changed? Policy, equipment, attitude, skills, knowledge? Again the facilitator asks individuals to generate ideas silently and then share them with the group for analysis and weighting. The study may stop at this point if no correctable factors are identified or if improvement action appears impractical or overly expensive. Again, careful topic selection would normally have eliminated studies aborted for these reasons.

In the majority of cases, the study proceeds and a written plan for improvement is prepared, defining terminology, outlining steps for change, and weighing estimated costs -- in terms of time and money --

against the benefit to be derived. Duties are assigned and dates for the beginning and end of the improvement action are decided. Choosing the improvement action marks the end of Stage 3. The specific steps for Stage 3 follow.

Outline for Stage 3
Definitive Assessment and Improvement Planning

A meeting of the original study team is called to present the findings of the study and plan for improvement. This meeting is scheduled to last about an hour and has the same facilitator as the Study Design Meeting.

Meeting Agenda for Stage 3

Definitive Assessment and Improvement Planning

(60 minutes)

Supplies needed: flipchart, wide felt-tipped pens, paper.

Presentation of Results

I. *Definitive Assessment (30 minutes)*

During this part of the meeting, which uses brainstorming rather than the nominal group process, the following procedure is used:

1. *Describing deficiencies*

The results of the assessment are presented to the study team. The team assesses these results.

2. *Generating correctable factors*

What are the possible causes amenable to change that contribute to the poor outcome? Put factors on the flipchart as the group presents them. Ask the group to consider:

a. Patient factors.

b. Provider factors.

c. Organizational factors.

d. Health environment factors

3. *Establishing priorities among correctable factors*

The facilitator can ask for priority weighting here as in Stage 1. Consideration of causality, correctability, and practicality should be considered when weighting the factors.

4. *Making a "go/no go" decision*

This will be based on group satisfaction that the most likely correctable factors have been identified.

II. *Planning Improvement Action* (30 minutes)

In this part of the meeting, the facilitator needs to do the following:

1. Establish the purpose of this phase, which is selecting the best improvement action for the correctable causative factor selected.

2. Generate improvement actions through simple brainstorminig or the nominal group technique. The facilitator writes down

suggested actions on a flipchart, whichever method is used. The group then discusses and weights the actions, usually by show of hands. A caution here is necessary: do not rush in and choose the first "obvious" improvement action. "Walk through" the actions via discussion, challenge them thoroughly, and examine them to determine whether they are the least expensive way to remedy the problem. Think about trying a less expensive action first, falling back on a more costly solution if the former does not appear workable.

3. Arrange the improvement actions in priority, according to weighting by the group. The top-weighted items usually are recommended as improvement actions. Lower priority improvement actions are recorded and retained for possible future use if the first choices prove ineffectual.

4. Record a "go/no go" decision by majority vote of the study team after establishing the following:

- What action will be undertaken?

- By whom?

- When?

- How long will the improvement phase last?

- What will be the estimated cost in time, effort, money? How do the likely gains stack up against the costs?

5. Take the decision, if it is "go," to administration for approval. This is the end of Stage 3.

Stage 4 — Improvement Action

Improvement action happens in the doing. The improvement action proceeds and may be monitored to be sure it is carried out properly.

Outline for Stage 4
Improvement Action

The purpose of this stage is to produce improvement in the particular health care problem already identified. The quality assurance coordinator or study team facilitator is responsible for directing improvement activities, organizing the effort, and obtaining necessary materials or personnel.

Stage 5 — Outcome Reassessment

The results of the improvement action are now assessed, using the same measurement tools as in Stage 2. The purpose of health accounting is to bring actual treatment results as close to the standard as possible through improvement action. To judge whether any change can be reasonably attributed to the improvement action, look for any other relevant factors that may have been introduced at the same time as the improvement action.

At this stage, if improvement action seems not to have been entirely successful, there may be a return to Stage 3 to initiate a new type of improvement planning, or it may be decided to continue the improvement action to see whether more time is required. On the other hand, if the improvement action achieves the MAS or comes reasonably close to it, it is judged successful. The results are fed into the overall quality assurance program of the facility and, if possible, published for wider dissemination.

Though the study is now concluded, there may be periodic monitoring to be certain the improvement is maintained. Completed health accounting studies may also inspire research and generate other studies, as well as serve as the basis for system changes within a facility.

Figure E shows the conclusion of the study referred to in Figure D. It gives the relationship between the MAS and the problem control rate before and after improvement action.

Noncontrol Rate

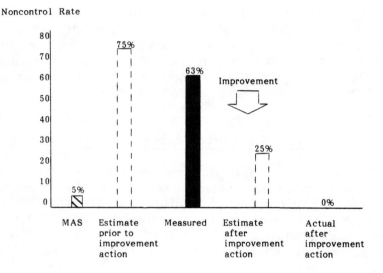

Figure E

Health Problem Noncontrol
Before and After Improvement Action

Definition of health problem noncontrol: patient (or family member) lacks knowledge of short-term rehabilitation goals.

Data showing improved outcomes provides feedback reinforcing health accounting activities. A problem-solving approach to patient care, looking at outcomes to be achieved, yields direct benefits to patients. There are also benefits to health professionals who, realizing they can make a difference, are challenged to continue improving the services they provide. A specific outline of steps for Stage 5 follows.

Outline for Stage 5
Outcome Reassessment

At the end of the improvement action study period, data are collected by the same method and for the same questions as were asked in Stage 2. The quality assurance coordinator may collect the data or delegate responsibility for its collection.

Outcome Reassessment Meeting (20 minutes)

This meeting is merely to set up procedures for collecting the reassessment data, following Stage 2 procedures. The same survey instrument is used, and either the same subjects as in Stage 2 or another sample from the same population base.

Implementing the Reassessment Plan

This means collection of the data as per the above, following the same procedures as before.

- Identify the sample.

- Contact the sample members via the appropriate method (phone, mail, in person, or via chart).

- Collect data with specialized survey instruments or tests.

- Continue until there is at least an 80 percent response rate.

Analyzing the Results

The quality assurance assistant or coordinator then compiles the sample results and calculates the *noncontrol rate. This data, showing whether or not the improvement action appears successful, are then presented to the study team.*

If the action proves successful, there will be a reduction of noncontrol of the problem to a level close to or below the MAS. The improvement action, of course, need not stop here, but may continue.

If the action is unsuccessful, there should be a return to Stage 3, and a reconvening of the study team. In rare cases, the MAS may be modified to a more realistic level.

In calculating the results of a study, it is useful to assess benefits achieved against costs. A study has both tangible and intangible costs and benefits.

Examples of tangible benefits would be improved patient outcomes, decreased length of patient stay, better reimbursement, and meeting JCAH standards. Intangible benefits could include better staff morale and improved community image of the facility. Supplies and staff time spent for the health accounting study would be some of the tangible costs. Staff irritation at having to conduct a study would be an example of intangible costs. Since the study topic was selected as one which would be cost effectively achievable, it is worth the time to assess, even roughly, how accurate the original judgments were about the efficiency of the study. Methods of trimming costs may become apparent in this exercise. For further information about cost effectiveness estimates, see Table 3, Improving the Impact of Occupational Therapy (AOTA, 1980).

A health accounting study performed in a clinic is kept on record for the JCAH. A copy is also forwarded to the central quality assurance committee, if there is one, and to hospital administration.

The study is over, but its influence may well continue in the form of permanent changes in procedure and heightened staff and patient morale. Occasional monitoring of outcomes should be repeated to see that results are maintained.

The next chapter describes a health accounting study conducted by occupational therapy students.

CHAPTER V

A STUDENT
HEALTH ACCOUNTING STUDY

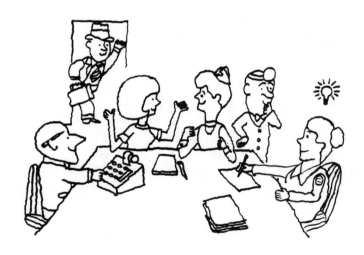

Health accounting is an interdisciplinary approach to a wide variety of problems.

V. A STUDENT
HEALTH ACCOUNTING STUDY

As part of their study of quality assurance, a group of thirty occupational therapy students were assigned to conduct a health accounting study. Their instructor continued to act as a resource person and instructed them via lecture, but it was basically the student's own "show." We will "walk through" their study here.

This student project actually took place, though certain details have been changed. The students decided to focus on improving aspects of their own education. Application of health accounting to a problem of this type is evidence of its versatility. Although the study stopped at Stage 3, it was a valuable exercise for the students.

Stage 1 -- Priority Setting

For the priority setting meeting, the class of 30 broke up into three priority setting teams of ten each. Each group of students rotated in the facilitator's job to give everyone experience. Group 1 will be followed below.

Introduction

The student acting as facilitator for the first part of the meeting clarified the purpose of the meeting, set the time-table, and reviewed ABNA and the nominal group technique. Introductions were unnecessary because the students already knew one another.

The three essential criteria for establishing priority problems -- importance, solvability, and cost effectiveness -- were written on the flipchart. The facilitator asked: "What problems in our educational program could we study that would meet the three criteria?"

Individual Topic Formulation

Each member of the group wrote topic ideas on a piece of blank paper. Going around the room twice, the facilitator for each group wrote down ideas on the flipchart without comment or discussion.

Group Collation and Discussion

The members of the first group taped up all their flipchart ideas on the classroom wall with masking tape. The facilitator asked them whether they understood each topic well enough to make a priority weighting. The students replied that they did.

Individual Topic Priority Weighting

Then they weighted the topics on a scale from one to five (see sample of Individual Priority Weighting Form, Appendix F).

Collation of Priority Weights

The weights were tallied for the group using a show of hands. These were then transferred to the Priority Topic Summary List (Appendix G).

Group Discussion and Reweighting of Topics

The group discussed the strong points and disadvantages of each topic. They used the form shown in Appendix E, Stage 1 Formulation of Topics, to describe their topics in more detail.

Three main topics emerged: (a) the problem of books unavailable to student library users, (b) the distraction of a square dance class taking place next door while occupational therapy students were attending lectures, and (c) the occupational therapy students' perception that they were unprepared for various clinical skills in fieldwork practice.

These topics were discussed. It was agreed that (b), the topic of the noisy dance class next door, could probably be handled by talking to the dance instructor or moving the occupational therapy class, without a need for elaborate planning of an improvement action. Topic (a) was shelved for the present.

Topic (c), the students' perceived lack of preparation for various elements of fieldwork practice, such as muscle testing, was given the highest weighting and chosen for final study by this group of students.

The three student groups came together to discuss their priority topics and topic (c) of the first group was chosen for study by all three groups.

Stage 2 — Initial Outcome Assessment

Literature Search

Each student participated in a coordinated literature search, bringing the findings to the study design meeting (next).

Study Team Selection and Study Design Meeting

The students broke up into three study design teams, all studying topic (c). As in Stage 1, they rotated in the facilitator's role. The students were not only team members, but were also the subjects of their study. They were assessing their own preparedness for clinical experience. The students followed the outline for the Study Design Meeting, breaking it into its component parts of "IDSAW" (Introduction, Design, Simulation, Analysis, and Wrap-up). Again, the facilitator's job was rotated. Here is how one student group conducted the study design meeting.

I -- Introduction. The facilitator clarified the purpose of the meeting, showed the place of Stage 2 in the five-stage system, and reviewed the reasons the topic was selected. Fieldwork preparation was important to the students and to the patients. The group felt their lack of preparation for fieldwork was an important problem, and solvable, with little cost involved. The students also presented the results of their literature search, but there was little directly relevant to their topic.

D -- Design. During the Design phase of the meeting, the students went over the following points:

1. Action Outcome Study
   The students determined that this was indeed an action outcome study, involving improvement of fieldwork preparation. The action causing the problem was the present classroom experience in various clinical skills students felt they would need during their fieldwork.

   This was not a decision outcome study, which might have dealt with decisions whether such training should have been provided in the first place. Clinical skills were already an accepted part of the curriculum, but the students still felt unprepared.

At the study design meeting, they refined the problem and described it more fully: student morale was low because they considered their clinical skills inadequate for starting their fieldwork experience. One of the student study design teams thought the problem was solvable through more in-class practice, using each other as stand-ins for patients, and through more observation of practicing occupational therapists. They felt, in summary, that the problem was important and solvable at little cost, and that its solution would prove of great benefit to themselves and their future patients.

Study Topic/Problem: Students feel clinical skills are inadequate for fieldwork experience.

2. Sample Size and Selection

Here the students reaffirmed that they and their classmates were the subjects of the study, i.e., the "patients." The providers, or people who needed to change, would be both themselves and their instructors.

The students used their class roster as the sample. Their whole class served as subjects making them a universe sample of thirty.

3. Defining Noncontrol of the Problem

The students decided that noncontrol of their problem meant being unprepared for fieldwork experience. This would be manifested by their lack of specific clinical skills, such as in muscle testing and ADL testing. They would not know what to do when asked to evaluate patients. Supervisors would find their techniques faulty.

One of the three student study design teams proposed two methods of determining noncontrol which were adopted by all class members. Each student would keep a self-assessment chart during the first days of the fieldwork experience, reporting when they felt unprepared for practicing a particular skill, as well as when they felt appropriately prepared for a task. Second, a performance evaluation report from clinical supervisors would be made for each student. It would evaluate how well the student performed the skills in question. The latter would be based on an interview questionnaire administered to clinical supervisors.

Therefore, there would be two measures of the problem of lack of preparedness. One was to be each student's self-assessment diary, the other the field supervisor's rating on each clinical task performed. Items in the diary would be scored on a five-point rating scale. The supervisor would score the same tasks using the same rating scale, with the lowest two scores constituting failure on that task.

4. Time-table
The students decided to study themselves as a universe sample when they began clinical fieldwork in one week's time and to conclude the study after finishing the first week of clinical.

Simulation. The students "walked through" their study in discussion and on paper. They set the MAS for both measures of problem noncontrol at 10 percent. That is, on all clinical tasks performed during the first week of fieldwork experience, not more than 10 percent of diary items could show failure and not more than 10 percent of field supervisor ratings on all tasks performed could show failure.

Their expected findings were that actual pre-improvement levels would be 66 percent on both measures, representing two-thirds of all fieldwork tasks, rather than the MAS of 10 percent. They estimated that after improvement action, their noncontrol rate would be reduced to as low as 5 percent. They felt it was possible to reach adequacy in the performance of almost all fieldwork tasks after improvement action. Their conclusions are summarized on the Stage 2 Study Design Form (Appendix H).

A -- Analysis. The students reviewed their study, which seemed practical and feasible. The gap between the MAS of 10 percent and their expected findings of 66 percent was 56 percent, leaving a large potential for improvement action, especially since they felt the MAS could be reduced to zero after improvement action. Therefore, a "go" decision was made to continue the study.

W -- Wrap-up. Duties were assigned and dates for completion set.

Study Implementation

To implement their study, each student kept a personal diary of the first week of fieldwork experience. They also interviewed supervisors about their own performance during that week.

In tabulating the results after that week, they learned to their surprise that, as far as supervisors were concerned, they were not inadequately prepared after all. In fact, they met the supervisors' expectations of adequate preparation, showing an average noncontrol rate of only 5 percent on all items, well below the MAS of 10 percent. If the supervisor ratings had been the sole measure of noncontrol, there would have been no need for improvement action.

However, the student self-evaluations told quite another story, reaching a noncontrol rate of 50 percent for all clinical tasks performed during the week. This discrepancy indicated that the students lacked confidence in their performance, even though supervisors gave them satisfactory ratings.

Stage 3 — Definitive Assessment and Improvement Planning

The results of the student study were presented to the class. The results indicated that actual fieldwork performance was not an aspect of the problem that needed remedy, since the class had more than reached the MAS. However, the students' lack of self-confidence in approaching fieldwork did require bolstering. Presentation of the study findings (see Figure F) on supervisors' evaluations proved a first step in that direction.

The students decided to go ahead with improvement planning even though the end of the semester was approaching.

Planning Improvement Action

The students devised a plan for increasing confidence in the areas of fieldwork included in the study. They planned to ask the instructors and university administration to schedule three curriculum hours for practicing fieldwork tasks on each other and for permitting class discussion of their anxieties. In addition, students would be assigned to observe experienced occupational therapists performing skills about which students felt unsure in the fieldwork setting before they themselves started. They recommended that students keep a diary to see whether a reduction in anxiety resulted. However, due to lack of time, the improvement action was never implemented; it was passed along to the next class, with recommendations that they complete the study.

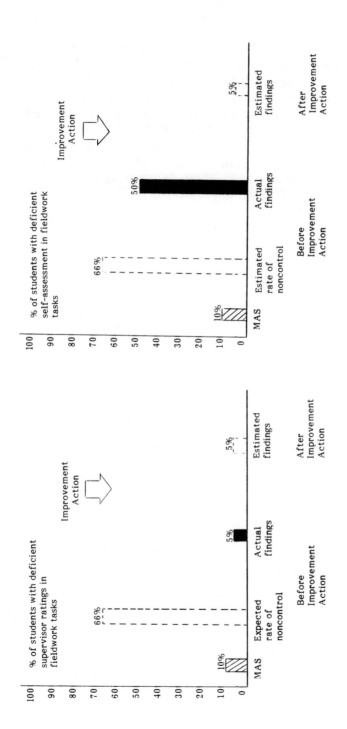

Figure F

Student Health Accounting Study

Through this example of a student study, and throughout this book, we have tried to give a succinct but complete overview of the application of health accounting to action outcomes. This manual serves as a stepping stone to the more comprehensive *Health Accounting for Quality Assurance* (Williamson, et al., 1981), referred to earlier, which gives the full range of procedures, including those for use with decision outcome studies. When readers have mastered what we have offered here, we urge them to move on and to broaden their range of skills.

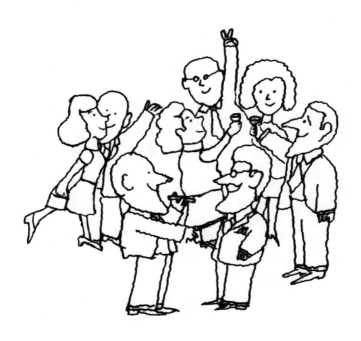

The end of a health accounting study marks the beginning of improved health, economic, or societal outcomes.

GLOSSARY OF TERMS

A

Achievable benefits not achieved (ABNA). Health care benefits presently attainable, but not being realized.

Action outcome. Results at any single point in time of carrying out a given decision.

D

Decision outcome. Results of a judgmental process regarding actions taken or not taken.

E

Efficacy. Achievable benefits of a health care intervention under ideal circumstances.

Effectiveness. Benefits achieved by a health care program under average or actual circumstances.

Efficiency. Extent to which desired outcomes are achieved with a minimum of unnecessary expenditure and effort.

H

Health accounting. A problem-oriented outcome approach to quality assurance designed to improve both effectiveness and efficiency of health care services.

Health care outcomes. Refers to any characteristic of patient, health problem, provider, or their interaction that results from health care received or withheld, measured at one point in time.

I

Improvement action. Implementation of educational programs, administrative policies, or other actions to change patient or practitioner behavior or health facility organization to effect health improvements, health risk reductions, or cost improvements.

J

Joint Commission on Accreditation of Hospitals (JCAH). A private organization representing a number of physicians' groups whose standards have become the preferred criteria for hospitals to demonstrate the quality of their services and thus be able to receive Medicare reimbursement.

M

Maximum acceptable standards (MAS). The highest percentage, consistent with quality care, of patients in the population studied whose health problem is out of control.

N

Nominal group process. A structured method of group decision making used in health accounting.

Q

Quality assurance (QA). The process of assessing and improving health care delivery.

S

Study design meeting. A meeting in Stage 2 of health accounting to plan initial outcome assessment and make a "go/no go" decision on the study plan.

BIBLIOGRAPHY

The American Occupational Therapy Association, Inc. *Standards of Practice for Occupational Therapy Services for the Developmentally Disabled Client, Standards of Practice for Occupational Therapy for Clients with Physical Disabilities, Standards of Practice for Occupational Therapy in a Home Health Program, and Standards of Practice for Occupational Therapy Services in a Mental Health Program,* Rockville, Maryland, The American Occupational Therapy Association, Inc., 1978.

The American Occupational Therapy Association, Inc. *Improving the Impact of Occupational Therapy,* Rockville, Maryland, The American Occupational Therapy Association, Inc., 1980.

Anderson, TP; et al. "Stroke Rehabilitation: Evaluation of Its Quality by Assessing Patient Outcomes," *Archives of Physical Medicine and Rehabilitation,* pp. 170–175, April 1978.

Codman, EA. "The Product of a Hospital," *Surgery, Gynecology, and Obstetrics,* April 1914, Vol. 18, pp. 491–496.

Commission on Accreditation of Rehabilitation Facilities. *Program Evaluation in Rehabilitation: Hospital Based Facilities,* Chicago, Illinois, Commission on Accreditation of Rehabilitation Facilities, May 1976.

Commission on Accreditation of Rehabilitation Facilities. *Program Evaluation: A First Step*, Chicago, Commission on Accreditation of Rehabilitation Facilities, November 1976.

Commission on Accreditation of Rehabilitation Facilities. *Program Evaluation in Vocational Rehabilitation Facilities*, Chicago, Illinois, Commission on Accreditation of Rehabilitation Facilities, July 1977.

Commission on Accreditation of Rehabilitation Facilities. *Program Evaluation in Work Activity Facilities*, Chicago, Illinois, Commission on Accreditation of Rehabilitation Facilities, January 1979.

Commission on Accreditation of Rehabilitation Facilities. *Program Evaluation in Inpatient Medical Rehabilitation Facilities*, Chicago, Illinois, Commission on Accreditation of Rehabilitation Facilities, December 1979.

Commission on Accreditation of Rehabilitation Facilities. *Program Evaluation in Outpatient Medical Rehabilitation Facilities*, Chicago, Illinois, Commission on Accreditation of Rehabilitation Facilities, February 1980.

Delbecq, AL; Van de Ven, AH; Gustafson, D. *Group Techniques for Program Planning: A Guide to Nominal Group and Delphi Processes*, Glenview, Illinois, Scott Foresman and Co., 1975.

Donabedian, A. *A Guide to Medical Care Administration*, New York, American Public Health Association, 1969.

Donabedian, A. *The Definition of Quality and Approaches to its Assessment*, Ann Arbor, Michigan, Health Administration Press, University of Michigan, 1980.

Donabedian, A. *The Criteria and Standards of Quality*, Ann Arbor, Michigan, Health Administration Press, University of Michigan, 1982.

Flexner, A. *Medical Education in the United States and Canada*, New York, Carnegie Foundation, Merrymount Press, 1910.

Garraway, WM; et al. "Management of Acute Stroke in the Elderly: Preliminary Results of a Controlled Trial," *British Medical Journal*, April 12, 1980.

Good, D. "Establishing an Effective Team Approach to and Throughout Treatment," Los Angeles, Daniel Freeman Hospital Medical Center, June 1981, Unpublished mimeograph.

Hopkins, H; Smith, H. *Willard and Spackman's Occupational Therapy*, 6th Edition, Philadelphia, JB Lippincott, 1983.

Holzemer, WL. "Research and Evaluation: An Overview," *Quality Review Bulletin*, March 1980.

Huxley, E. *Florence Nightingale*, New York, Putnam, 1975.

The Joint Commission on Accreditation of Hospitals. *The QA Guide*, Chicago, Illinois, The Joint Commission on Accreditation of Hospitals, 1980.

The Joint Commission on Accreditation of Hospitals. *Accreditation Manual for Hospitals*, 1982 Edition, Chicago, Illinois, The Joint Commission on Accreditation of Hospitals, 1981.

Kuntavanish, A; Ostrow, PC. "The Outcomes of Back Conservation Education," *Quality Review Bulletin*, April 1980.

Ostrow, PC; Kaufman, K. "Improved Productivity in an Acute-Care Psychiatric Occupational Therapy

Program: A Quality Assurance Study," *Productivity Improvements in Physical and Occupational Therapies*, Chicago, Illinois, The American Hospital Association, 1981.

Ostrow, PC. "The Historical Precedents for Quality Assurance in Health Care," *The American Journal of Occupational Therapy*, Vol. 37, No. 1, pp. 23-26, January 1983a.

Ostrow, PC. "Quality Assurance Requirements of The Joint Commission on Accreditation of Hospitals," *The American Journal of Occupational Therapy*, Vol. 37, No. 1, pp. 27-31, January 1983b.

Van de Ven, AH; Delbecq, AL. "Nominal Versus Interacting Group Processes for Committee Decision-Making Effectiveness," *The Academy of Management Journal*, No. 2, pp. 203-212, June 1971.

Williamson, JW; Aronovitch, S; Simonson, L; Ramirez, C; Kelly, D. "Health Accounting: An Outcome-Based System of Quality Assurance: Illustrative Application to Hypertension," *Bulletin of the New York Academy of Medicine*, 51(6):727-738, June 1975.

Williamson, JW. *Assessing and Improving Health Care Outcomes: The Health Accounting Approach to Quality Assurance*, Cambridge, Ballinger Publishing Company, 1978a.

Williamson, JW. "Formulating Priorities for Quality Assurance Activity," *Journal of The American Medical Association*, 139(7):631-637, February 1978b.

Williamson, JW. "Outcome-Based Quality Assurance Gets a Scorecard," *Group Practice*, May-June 1978c.

Williamson, JW; Braswell, HR; Horn, SD; Lohmeyer, S. "Priority Setting in Quality Assurance: Reliability of Staff Judgments in Medical Institutions," *Medical Care*, 16(3):931-940, November 1978d.

Williamson, JW; Braswell, HR; Horn, SD; "Validity of Medical Staff Judgments in Establishing Quality Assurance Priorities," *Medical Care*, 17(4):331–346, April 1979.

Williamson, JW; Goldschmidt, P; Jillson, I. *Medical Practice Information Demonstration Project*, Final Report, Contract 282-77-0068GS, Office of the Assistant Secretary for Health, Department of Health, Education and Welfare, Policy Research Incorporated, Baltimore, 1980.

Williamson, JW; Ostrow, PC; Braswell, HR. *Health Accounting for Quality Assurance: A Manual for Assessing and Improving the Outcomes of Care*, Rockville, Maryland, The American Occupational Therapy Association, Inc., 1981.

Williamson, JW. *Principles of Quality Assurance and Cost Containment in Health Care*, San Francisco, Jossey-Bass, 1982a.

Williamson, JW, et al. *Teaching Quality Assurance and Cost Containment*, San Francisco, Jossey-Bass, 1982b.

APPENDIX A

Skills Development Exercise I -- Definitions

Answer Key

1. The efficacy of this splint is 98 percent (clinical trial rate). The current effectiveness in the clinic is 50 percent. On the question of efficiency, the cheaper splint would be preferable.

2. The MAS is 10 percent.

APPENDIX B

Answers depend on the situation and group judgment as to which element, decision, or action is most important.

1. <u>Decision</u>. The decision to refer to occupational therapy is the crux of the problem as stated.

2. <u>Action</u>. Improved therapeutic management seems to be at issue. Concern about adequate diagnosis is not mentioned.

3. <u>Decision</u>. Judgment about whether to send patients to rehabilitation is at issue here.

4. <u>Both</u>. Which patients to educate and how to do it successfully; both decision and action seem to be at issue.

5. <u>Action</u>. Better communication and coordination are the required actions.

6. <u>Decision</u>. The decision by therapists about which patients should have sensory integrative therapy is the problem.

APPENDIX C

Skills Development Exercise 3

Selecting Study Sample and Measuring Action Outcomes

Answer Key

There is no single "correct" set of answers for these problems. Here are some samples:

1a. All stroke patients, admitted to the hospital in one year as listed in medical records.

b. A retrospective sample, approximately 35 patients, starting with the latest discharge and consecutively sampling patient records for the past three months.

c. Measure number of days between admission and referral.

2a. All hospitalized nonambulatory patients receiving occupational therapy.

b. Every other patient selected from patients' concurrent daily roster until 30 are included in the sample, providing the current month is representative of all months.

c. Measure the number of canceled or late treatments due to break-downs in the transportation system for these 30 patients until they are discharged or until one month is over. Record the number of timely transports also for this sample.

3a.   All rehabilitation patients and families.

b.   A one out of every four, two-month, concurrent sample of patients and significant others about to receive the four-hour stress management training in occupational therapy.

c.   Survey patients' and family members' knowledge of stress management techniques before occupational therapy and by phone 60 days post-discharge to determine effects of stress management training program.

APPENDIX D

Stage 2 Study Design Summary

(based on Study Design Meeting)

Facility:_____Date:_____

<u>Introduction</u>

Study Topic: _____

<u>Design</u>

Which Type of Study?

Decision outcomes _____

Action outcomes _____
(for this <u>Primer,</u> it is assumed an action outcome
study will be done).

Who and What to Study?

Describe the population from which the sample
will be drawn (age, sex, diagnosis, or health
problem, etc.).

_____

_____

Estimate Annual Size of Population_____

Where to Locate Subjects?

Describe the source or location for the population to be measured (appointment lists, charts,
etc.) _____

_____

Describe Sample Method (consecutive, random,
etc.) and Interval (one in three for three months,
universe, etc.). _____

_____

Sample Size Estimated _____(25 recommended minimum)

How to Measure Outcomes?

Action outcomes

Describe noncontrol of the problem (what
objective, measurable phenomenon tells
you the problem is out of control?).

_____

_____

Describe noncontrol measure _____

_____

_____

_____

_____

Simulation (likely results of the assessment estimated to determine feasibility).

	Expected Findings Pre-Improvement	Maximum Acceptable Standards (MAS)	Expected Findings Post-Improvement
	(1)	(2)	(3)

Action Outcomes:

Noncontrol Rate (out of 100%)	____ %	____ %	____ %

Analysis

Decide if estimated benefits outweigh estimated costs.

Yes_____   No_____

Wrap-up

Assignments for Study Completion

_____

_____

_____

_____

_____

APPENDIX E

Stage 1 Formulation of Topics

Institution: *University X*   Date: *4/10/82*

	Topic A	Topic B	Topic C
Subject/Setting Characteristics			
Identify subjects/patients involved in this problem -- age? location? sex?	Student library users	Students attending lectures in Room A	All Occupational therapy students who are ready for fieldwork
Health Problem Characteristics			
What diagnosis or deficiencies define the patients involved. Arthritis? ADL deficiencies?	Not applicable	Not applicable	Not applicable
Provider/Facility Characteristics			
Who would need to change to improve outcomes?	University Librarian	Room B dance instructor	University Professors in Occupational Therapy curriculum
Possible change to improve outcomes			
What change is necessary to improve outcomes. (Note the overall change, not the many possible ways to achieve it)	Improve availability of books (obtain more copies, keep shorter check-out schedule)	Reduce noise in Room B (move class to new location, turn down phonograph)	Increase students' clinical skill and/or confidence in preparation for fieldwork experience (review and practice of clinical skills just prior to fieldwork)

APPENDIX F

Individual Priority Weighting Form

Institution: _University X_ _____ Date: _4/10/82_

Instructions:

1. Using a scale of 1 through 5 (5 = high), weight the potential improvement for the target benefit (such as health) that might be achieved within acceptable resource constraints (such as cost and time).

2. After group analysis of topics, record your second item weight in the right column.

Collation Topic	Initial Weights	Revised Weights	Collation Topic	Initial Weights	Revised Weights
A	4	3	K		
B	4	2	L		
C	5	5	M		
D			N		
E			O		
F			P		
G			Q		
H			R		
I			S		
J			T		

APPENDIX G

Priority Topic Summary List

Institution: _University X_   Date: _4/10/82_

Topic	Initial Weight	Total	Second Weight	Total
A Assuring the availability in the University library of books assigned as reading in occupational therapy classes.	WT: 5│4│3│2│1 = #: 1│1│5│2│2	30	WT: 5│4│3│2│1 = #: 1│1│3│3│3	27
B Decreasing the noise level from a classroom adjoining the occupational therapy classroom.	WT: 5│4│3│2│1 = #: 0│1│2│3│4	20	WT: 5│4│3│2│1 = #: 0│0│1│3│6	15
C Improving the confidence and/or level of skill of occupational therapy students in performing clinical skills.	WT: 5│4│3│2│1 = #: 5│2│1│1│1	39	WT: 5│4│3│2│1 = #: 6│3│1│0│0	45
D	WT: 5│4│3│2│1 = #: │ │ │ │		WT: 5│4│3│2│1 = #: │ │ │ │	

#Refers to the number of persons assigning this weight. Again, only Topics A, B, and C are shown here.

98

APPENDIX H

Stage 2 Study Design Summary

(based on Study Design Meeting)

Facility: _University X_   Date: _5/10/82_

Introduction

Study Topic: _Better preparation during the academic year; second year OT students don't feel ready to practice clinical skills._

Design

Which Type of Study?

    Decision outcome _____

    Action outcome _____✓_____
(for this <u>Primer</u>, it is assumed an action outcome study will be done).

Who and What to Study?

    Describe the population from which the sample will be drawn (age, sex, diagnosis, or health problem, etc.).

    All OT students in the class, ages

    _18 - 32_

Estimate Annual Size of Population ___30___

Where to Locate Subjects?

Describe the source or location for the population to be measured (appointment lists, charts, etc.) _____

_____Class roster_____

Describe Sample Method (consecutive, random, etc.) and Interval (one in three for three months, universe, etc.). _____

_____Universe_____

Sample Size Estimated ___30___ (25 recommended minimum)

How to Measure Outcomes?

Action outcomes

Describe noncontrol of the problem (what objective, measurable phenomenon tells you the problem is out of control?).

Student feelings of unpreparedness and lack of

preparation for fieldwork as observed by supervisors.

Describe noncontrol measure _Skills_

performed, recorded in student self-

assessment diary and by supervisor

questionnaires at the end of each

fieldwork day.

Simulation (likely results of the assessment estimated to determine feasibility).

	Expected Findings Pre-Improvement	Maximum Acceptable Standards (MAS)	Expected Findings Post-Improvement
	(1)	(2)	(3)
Action Outcomes:			
Noncontrol Rate (out of 100%)	66 %	10 %	5 %

(for both noncontrol measures)

Analysis

Decide if estimated benefits outweigh estimated costs.

Yes __✓__   No_____

Wrap-up

Assignments for Study Completion

Students will keep a self-assessment diary; will ask supervisors to rate them according to questionnaire.

_____

_____

INDEX

ABOUT THE AUTHORS

Patricia C. Ostrow, MA, OTR, is Director of the Quality Assurance Division of The American Occupational Therapy Association, Inc., and has taught patient care evaluation for more than seven years. Ms. Ostrow chaired the Liaison Network of Health Care Practitioners other than Physicians which advised the National Professional Standards Review Council. In collaboration with Dr. Williamson, she implemented three health accounting demonstrations in occupational therapy settings. She also developed and conducted a series of nationwide seminars on health accounting for members of the Association. She is a co-author of the *Health Accounting for Quality Assurance* manual and numerous other writings on quality assurance.

John W. Williamson, MD, is a Professor of Health Services Administration and International Health at the Johns Hopkins School of Hygiene and Public Health. Dr. Williamson originated the concepts and procedures of health accounting and is a contributing editor to The Joint Commission on Accreditation of Hospitals' *QA Guide.* His research has established the reliability, validity, feasibility, and practicality of using health accounting in multiple and varied health care settings. He has served as a consultant to many groups, including the National Academy of Science, Institute of Medicine, and the National Center for Health Services Research and Development. Dr. Williamson has written numerous books and articles in the health care field.

Barbara E. Joe, MA, is a Technical Writer in the Quality Assurance Division of The American Occupational Therapy Association, Inc. She has many years of experience in public policy development and has published works in a variety of health and human service fields.